I0830468

The Obesity Home Remedy Manual

How To Make Changes That Fit Your Lifestyle To Beat Obesity

By

Rusty R. Miranda

Disclaimer:

The information in this book is provided solely for educational purposes and is not intended to substitute for professional medical advice. The reader should check with their physician to see if the information applies to their situation because everyone is different.

Table Of Contents

Introduction:

The specialty of medication is very curious. Sometimes, clinical medicines become laid out that don't work. Despite their lack of effectiveness, these treatments are passed down from one generation of doctors to the next through sheer inertia and survive for a surprising amount of time.

Think about the restorative utilization of bloodsuckers (dying) or, say, routine tonsillectomy. Unfortunately, one such example is obesity treatment. A person's body mass index, which is calculated by dividing their weight in kilograms by the square of their height in meters, is used to define obesity.

Obesity is characterized by an excessive accumulation of body fat, which results in declining health, disability, and an increase in mortality and morbidity. An individual's weight is not entirely set in stone to be in the fat reach when the individual's weight file (BMI) is 30.0 kg/m2 or higher for most non-Asian populaces.Obesity is a multifaceted, long-time period circumstance characterized with the aid of using immoderate frame fats and sometimes terrible fitness due to more than one factors. Naturally, extra frame fats now no longer motivate disease. But when you have an excessive amount of greater fats to your body, it could alternate the way it works.These adjustments are gradual, can worsen over time, and may have poor consequences on health.

There are many ways that obesity affects your body. Some are just the mechanical effects of having more fat on your body. For instance, you can define a reasonable boundary between additional load on your body and additional tension on your skeleton and joints. Chemical changes in your blood that raise your risk of diabetes, heart disease, and stroke are another less obvious effect.

There are still some unclear effects. Obesity, for instance, is associated with an increased risk of certain cancers. Obesity is statistically associated with an increased risk of all causes of premature death. The good news is that you can reduce your health risks by losing some of your excess body fat. Studies have shown that even a modest weight loss of 5 to 10 percent can significantly reduce these risks.Your fitness may be extensively tormented by even the smallest weight changes. Few out of every odd weight reduction technique works for everybody. The majority of human beings have attempted to shed pounds a couple of times. And maintaining the weight loss is just as important as losing it.

Chapter 1:

Symptoms And Causes Of Obesity

Here are some symptoms of obesity. These include:

- Back and joint pain,
- Feeling isolated,
- Snoring,
- Feeling constantly tired, and not being able to exercise.
- Increased sweating is also a sign of obesity.

The Root Causes Of Obesity

Obesity is a complex problem with many reasons. It occurs when the body stores more calories as fat.
If you consume a lot of energy—especially from foods high in fat and sugar—but don't use all of it by doing physical activity, a lot of the extra energy will be stored as fat in your body.

Calories: Calories are the units by which food's energy value is measured. To maintain a healthy weight, the average physically active man requires approximately 2,500 calories per day, and the average physically active woman requires approximately 2,000 calories per day.

Although this number sounds high, consuming certain types of food can help you reach it. For instance, eating a hugely important point burger, fries, and a milkshake can add up to 1,500 calories - and that is only 1 feast.

As well as this, many individuals don't meet the suggested active work levels for grown-ups, so the abundance of calories consumed turns out to be put away as fat in the body.

Diet: Obesity is caused by several factors, including diet, lifestyle, and other factors. The most typical ones include:

- Eating a lot of processed or fast food, which has a lot of fat and sugar,
- Drinking too much alcohol, which has a lot of calories,
- Eating a lot of food cooked in a restaurant, which may have a lot of fat and sugar, Eating more than you need,

- Drinking too many sugary drinks, like soft drinks and fruit juice,
- Comfort eating, which some people do because they have a low self-esteem or mood.

A healthy diet has also become more challenging as a result of changes in society. Food with a lot of calories is being heavily advertised and promoted because it is cheaper and easier to prepare.

Active work: The absence of active work is one more significant component connected with corpulence. Many jobs require workers to spend the majority of their time at a desk. They also drive rather than walk or ride a bicycle.
Many people rarely exercise regularly and prefer to watch television, play computer games, or browse the internet for relaxation.

If you don't exercise enough, your body stores the extra energy you consume as fat and doesn't use the energy from food.

Adults should engage in at least 150 minutes of weekly moderate-intensity aerobic activity, such as fast walking or cycling, according to the Department of Health and Social Care.   This needn't bother with being done all in a solitary meeting, however, can be separated into more modest periods. You could, for instance, exercise for 30 minutes five days a week.

If you're living with stoutness and attempting to shed pounds, you might have to do more activity than this. Starting small and gradually increasing your weekly exercise routine may be beneficial.

Genetics: Some genes are linked to being overweight and obese. Genes may have an impact on how the body converts food into energy and stores fat in some people. Qualities can likewise influence individuals' way of life decisions.
There are likewise a few uncommon hereditary circumstances that can cause corpulence, like Prader-Willi disorder.

Although having a large appetite, for example, is one of your parents' genetic characteristics, it is not impossible to lose weight.

Obesity is frequently more closely associated with environmental factors, such as a lack of easy access to healthy food or childhood eating habits.

Medical reasons: In some instances, weight gain may be caused by underlying medical conditions. These are some:

- An underactive thyroid organ (hypothyroidism) - where your thyroid organ doesn't deliver an adequate number of chemicals
- Cushing's condition - is an intriguing issue that causes the overproduction of steroid chemicals.

However, if these conditions are correctly diagnosed and treated, they should make it easier to lose weight.

Weight gain can be caused by taking certain medications, such as some steroids, diabetes, epilepsy, and mental illness medications, such as some antidepressants and schizophrenia medications.

Age: Obesity can affect anyone, even young children, at any age. However, hormonal shifts and a less active lifestyle as you get older raise your risk of obesity. Additionally, as you get older, your body's muscle mass tends to decrease. By and large, lower bulk prompts a reduction in digestion. Additionally, these modifications can make it harder to lose weight and reduce calorie requirements. You will probably put on weight as you get older if you don't consciously control what you eat and increase your physical activity.

Chapter 2:

Obesity's Hormonal Causes

Hormones are chemicals that tell our bodies how to do things. They are considered to cause stoutness. Appetite, metabolism (the rate at which our body burns kilojoules for energy), and body fat distribution are all influenced by the hormones leptin, insulin, sex hormones, and growth hormone. These hormones have degrees that inspire strange metabolism and the buildup of frame fat in overweight individuals.

The endocrine system is a collection of glands that inject hormones into our bloodstream. Our body is assisted in coping with various events and stresses by the endocrine system, which collaborates with the nervous system and immune systems. Obesity can result from excess or deficiency of hormones, and obesity can result in hormonal changes.

Leptin and obesity: The hormone leptin is secreted into our bloodstream and is produced by fat cells. A person's appetite is reduced by leptin by acting on specific brain centers to suppress the desire to eat. It likewise appears to control how the body deals with its store of muscle versus fat.

People with obesity tend to have higher levels of leptin than people with normal weight because leptin is made from fat. Be that as it may, regardless of having more elevated levels of this hunger-decreasing chemical, individuals who are corpulent aren't as delicate with the impacts of leptin and, subsequently, tend not to feel full during and after a feast. Why obese people's brains aren't receiving leptin messages is the subject of ongoing research.

Obesity and insulin: Insulin is a hormone produced by the pancreas that regulates the metabolism of fat and carbohydrates. Insulin encourages fat, muscles, and the liver to absorb glucose (sugar) from the blood. In order to ensure that energy is available for day-to-day activities and to maintain normal levels of circulating glucose, this is an essential process.

Obesity can lead to the loss of insulin signals and the inability of tissues to regulate glucose levels. The development of metabolic syndrome and type II diabetes may result from this.

Corpulence and sex chemicals: Muscle versus fat conveyance assumes a significant part in the improvement of weight-related conditions like coronary illness, stroke, and a few types of joint pain. Fat around our midsection is a higher gamble factor for infection than fat put away on our base, hips, and thighs. It appears to be that estrogens and androgens help to conclude muscle-to-fat ratio conveyance. Estrogens are sex chemicals made by the ovaries in premenopausal ladies. Every menstrual cycle, they are responsible for triggering ovulation.

Testicles and ovaries in men and postmenopausal women do not produce a lot of estrogens. All things being equal, a large portion of their estrogen is created in their muscle-to-fat ratio, in spite of the fact that at much lower sums than what is delivered in premenopausal ovaries. The testicles produce a lot of androgens in younger men. These levels gradually decrease as a man ages.

Body fat distribution shifts are linked to changes in sex hormone levels as men and women get older. Women of childbearing age tend to store fat in their lower body in a "pear-shaped" pattern, whereas older men and women who have gone through menopause tend to store fat around their abdomen in an "apple-shaped" pattern. Postmenopausal ladies who are taking estrogen supplements don't collect fat around their midsection. Creature studies have likewise shown that an absence of estrogen prompts unnecessary weight gain.

Weight and development chemical: The pituitary organ in our cerebrum produces a development chemical, which impacts an individual's level and helps fabricate bone and muscle. Metabolism, or the rate at which we burn kilojoules for energy, is also influenced by growth hormones. Growth hormone levels in obese individuals are lower than in people of normal weight, according to researchers.

Obesity and inflammation factor: Fat tissue low-grade chronic inflammation is also linked to obesity. Inflammatory factors and obesity Excessive fat storage causes stress reactions in fat cells, which in turn causes the fat cells and immune cells in the adipose (fat) tissue to release proinflammatory factors.

Hormones associated with obesity as a disease risk factor: Obesity is linked to a higher risk of cardiovascular disease, stroke, and several types of cancer, as well as a lower quality of life and shorter lifespan. For instance, the expanded creation of estrogens in the fat of more seasoned ladies who are corpulent is related to an expansion in bosom disease risk, demonstrating that the wellspring of estrogen creation is significant.

Hormones and obesity behavior: Obese people have high levels of hormones that encourage fat storage. Over time, it appears that overeating and not getting enough exercise "reset" the processes that control appetite and the distribution of body fat, making the person physiologically more likely to gain weight. The body resists short-term disruptions like crash dieting because it is constantly trying to keep its equilibrium.

Different investigations have shown that an individual's blood leptin level drops after a low-kilojoule diet. Lower leptin levels might expand an individual's craving and dial back their digestion. This might assist with making sense of why crash calorie counters ordinarily recapture their shed pounds. Although more research is required before this becomes a reality, it is possible that leptin therapy will one day assist dieters in maintaining their weight loss over the course of time.

There is proof to propose that drawn-out conduct changes, like smart dieting and standard activity, can control the body to shed an abundance of muscle versus fat and keep it off. Bariatric surgery or healthy eating and exercise have also been shown to improve insulin resistance, reduce inflammation, and help regulate obesity hormones, according to studies. Additionally, losing weight is linked to a lower risk of heart disease, stroke, type II diabetes, and some cancers.

Chapter 3:

Five Steps to Structure a Long-Term Obesity Treatment

Obesity treatment aims to achieve and maintain a healthy weight. This works on general well-being and brings down the gamble of creating complexities connected with weight.

You might have to work with a group of well-being experts — including a dietitian, conduct guide, or a stoutness-trained professional — to help you comprehend and make changes in your eating and movement propensities.

Typically, the initial goal of treatment is a modest weight loss of 5 to 10 percent of your total weight. That means that assuming you weigh 200 pounds (91 kilograms), you'd have to lose something like 10 to 20 pounds (4.5 to 9 kilograms) for your well-being to start to get to the next level. However, the advantages increase with weight loss.

All health improvement plans require changes in your dietary patterns and expanded active work. The severity of your obesity, your overall health, and your willingness to follow your weight-loss plan will determine the best treatment options for you.

1. Why do I weigh so much?

Regardless of what you could pursue, the issue of corpulence isn't brought about by any single food and it's not only an issue of 'an absence of resolve'. Many variables impact what we eat, truth be told. Since our lifestyles and environment have changed over the past few decades, it can be difficult to make healthy choices and we tend to eat more ready-made or takeout meals. When compared to meals prepared at home, this typically results in more fat, sugar, and salt, as well as larger portions.

At the same time, we are not moving as much as previous generations. Our positions and relaxation exercises are bound to include plunking down, and we're more averse to walking or by bike. Additionally, since many of us are now working from home more, we have missed out on the chance to exercise on the way to work.

You can lower your risk of heart and circulatory disease by as much as 35% by getting more active. As a result, we need to be careful about what we eat and how we exercise. This frequently entails making an effort to eat healthfully despite our busy schedules and finding ways to fit exercise into our schedules.

Consider the reasons why you might have gained weight as a good first step. Is this a recent alteration or an ongoing pattern? When you started gaining weight, did you start doing something different, like eating out more, being less active, or eating different foods?

Try recording what you eat with a diet tracker app on your smartphone or keeping a food and drink diary for a week in a notebook if you're not sure where you're going wrong.

2. Set a goal for yourself to lose weight.

It will be so difficult to lose weight. Determine how much weight you need to lose first. With additional individuals becoming overweight, how we view a 'solid weight' can become slanted.

Your weight concerning your height is measured by your body mass index (BMI). A free online tool can help you determine your BMI and the ideal weight if you know these measurements.

Don't feel like you have to do anything extreme if you weigh more than you think you do. Separate it into little objectives and spotlight on it with extra care.

Try to lose 10% of your body weight if you have a lot of weight to lose. Even if you end up being overweight, this will have significant health benefits and may seem more doable. If it takes a long time to reach your ideal weight, don't get discouraged. It probably took a long time for it to start coming on slowly.

3. Make the change that fit your lifestyle

Diets, tools, and foods that claim to help us lose weight are plentiful. Despite these baffling decisions, the fundamental standard of shedding pounds is basic: Calories must be consumed at a lower rate than energy expended.

Beyond that, each person's ideal diet will differ, and sticking to a plan is one of the most important factors. Finding the right path for you is the most important thing.

Many people find it helpful to avoid thinking of a "diet" and instead focus on a long-term strategy that works with their lifestyle. Certain individuals find diminishing fat or sugars works, some count calories, while others bring down their calorie consumption on specific days. To ensure that you don't miss out on vital nutrients, make sure your plan doesn't omit whole food groups.

Consider what will work best for you if you live with someone else and need their support to avoid being tempted to eat unhealthy foods at home. This means being honest about your lifestyle, like how much you can afford to eat, how well you cook, and what you like to eat.

You must make permanent changes to see a change in your weight that lasts, so make sure these are realistic. Little changes can feel immaterial, however, they add up bit by bit, assuming you stick to them.

To avoid being tempted by unhealthy foods at home, it can be crucial to have someone else's support if you live with them. You can even ask them to help you lose weight or support you.

Bunch support functions admirably for certain individuals. There is some evidence that those who join a slimming group lose more weight than those who don't. It very well may merit conversing with your GP or practice nurture, who will want to let you know if there are neighborhood bunches you can join or be alluded to, and they might have the option to offer you other help, as well.

A mix of diet changes and getting more dynamic has been demonstrated to be more viable than simply changing what you eat, so ponder ways of getting more dynamic. That could be going for a walk or a bike ride rather than driving, working out at home, or going for a walk or a run with a friend. If 150 minutes of exercise per week seems like a lot at first, break it up into 10-minute sessions.

Make an effort not to depend on practice as your main weight reduction system: It will benefit your heart health if you do more of it without changing your diet, but it won't likely help you lose weight.

4. Eat a decent eating routine

Decreased calorie, low-calorie, or light adaptations of your number one food sources might be useful, yet don't expect this to imply that they are additionally low in salt and sugar. Therefore, read food labels and try to make healthy choices rather than just lower-calorie ones.

Keeping up with even a little weight reduction is helpful for your well-being in the long haul and something to be glad for

You don't have to remove all food varieties that are higher in calories - some of them accompany solid supplements, for instance, sleek fish, unsalted nuts, and avocado. But you might want to eat them less often or limit how much you eat.

5. Don't give up if your progress is slow.

Reaching your "ideal" weight can take some time and sometimes seem impossible. If your weight loss is sluggish or you reach a plateau, don't get discouraged. Maintaining even a modest weight loss is something to be proud of and good for your health in the long run. Thus, carry on!

Way Of Life And Home Cures

Your work to conquer stoutness is bound to find success assuming that you follow procedures at home notwithstanding your conventional treatment plan. Some examples include:

Finding out about your condition: You can learn more about why you developed obesity and what you can do about it by getting educated about it. You might feel more able to take charge of your treatment and stick to your plan. Consider discussing reputable self-help books with your doctor or therapist.

Establishing attainable objectives: When you need to lose a lot of weight, you might set unattainable goals like trying to lose too much weight too quickly.

Avoid putting yourself at risk of failure: Put forth every day or week-by-week objectives for exercise and weight reduction. Instead of making drastic changes to your diet that you won't likely be able to maintain over time, try making small adjustments.

Adherence to your treatment regimen: It can be challenging to alter a way of life that you may have followed for several years. Be straightforward with your PCP, advisor, or other medical care experts if you find your action or eating objectives slipping. You can collaborate to develop novel strategies or concepts.

Obtaining assistance: Get the support of your loved ones to reach your weight loss goals. Encircle yourself with individuals who will uphold you and help you, not damage your endeavors. Ensure they comprehend how significant weight reduction is to your well-being. You might also want to join a support group for losing weight.

Maintaining a record: Maintain a food and activity diary. You can use this record to help you keep track of what you eat and how much you exercise. You can figure out what works well for you and what might be holding you back. You can also use your log to keep track of other important health parameters like your fitness level, blood pressure, and cholesterol levels.

Chapter 4:

The Diet Plan For Obesity

Foods to Eat on an Obesity Diet:
Here are some foods to include in your plan to lose weight:

1. Vitamins and fiber:

Vitamins and fiber can be found in abundance in fruits. Numerous studies show a link between eating more fruits and losing weight, probably because fruits are high in fiber. Additionally, eating foods high in fiber helps you stay full longer. Moreover, organic products have a bogus standing in that they don't assist in losing weight since they contain sugar, yet this sugar is regular and makes no mischief to the human body.

2. Vegetables with Vitamins and Antioxidants:

A few examinations have found that individuals who eat more verdant green vegetables over the long run shed pounds. Vegetables like spinach, broccoli, and so on. have loads of calcium and fiber that additionally help in fat consumption.

3. Vegetables And Beans:

Vegetables and beans are awesome to remember for veggie-lover diet plans or plant-based diet plans. Likewise, a rich wellspring of protein. They are exceptionally nutritious, which makes them an ideal staple in any eating regimen. They can help you feel full and eat less because they have a lot of protein and fiber in them. This helps you lose weight over time.

Examples of popular beans and legumes include:

Peanuts, chickpeas, black beans, soybeans, kidney beans, and lentils are the others.

4. Low-Fat Dairy:

Dairy food sources like milk, cheddar, eggs, curd, and so forth. contain rich measures of protein and bunches of fundamental nutrients like calcium. The majority of Indian diets include fresh, low-fat yogurt or curd to improve gut health. Additionally, cottage cheese can be included because it supplies the body with energy. Dairy consumption was found to reduce belly fat, inflammation, and the risk of type 2 diabetes, among other things, in one study. In this way, consuming dairy items in moderate amounts is correct.

5. Lean Protein:

Consuming a diet high in protein has been shown to lower levels of the hunger-inducing hormone ghrelin and increase levels of the satiating hormone peptide YY. These hormones have a powerful effect on your body.

Additionally, the human body gains muscle and strength from lean protein. Salmon, chicken, and other proteins are included in this category. Because they contain less saturated fat, these foods are recommended. Saturated fat, which raises cholesterol levels and poses other health risks, is found in greater quantities in red meats like lamb, pork, and beef.

Food Sources To Keep Away From In a Weight Diet Plan

Thus, here sharing a rundown of food sources to stay away from in a heftiness diet plan:

- Burgers, pizza, and fries are all examples of fast food.
- Chips, pakoras, and samosas are all deep-fried foods.

- Sweets like mithai and gulab jamun, among other things.
- Sugar-sweetened beverages, alcoholic beverages, and sodas are examples of processed foods that contain a lot of fat and carbohydrates.

While obesity is a growing health issue in many nations, it has recently spread to India as well. technological advancements, AI's introduction, etc. are all indications that humans are changing daily.

However, our health is in jeopardy as a result of our hustle. Our eating habits and way of life have changed significantly as a result of the convenience of food-ordering apps. We are all, without a doubt, well aware of the dangers and issues that come with being overweight or obese. As a result, more people are looking for a diet plan to help them lose weight.

In addition to the fact that being overweight or obese can have an impact on one's quality of life, it is also known that it contributes to several chronic diseases like Type 2 diabetes, high cholesterol, heart disease, and others. In this way, we should comprehend how we can handle corpulence through a sound eating routine and roll out compelling improvements in our way of life.

Test Diet Plan For Stout Individuals

Here I'm sharing an essential rule as far as where to begin arranging your eating routine. As a result, you can use this sample to determine what works for you and what doesn't.

Breakfast: Aloe vera juice, unsweetened milk, coffee, or tea, along with toast, eggs, porridge, oatmeal, or beetroot oats chilla.

Lunch: salad + entire wheat roti + vegetables + earthy colored rice + dal

Evening: Fruits, nuts, and green tea for

dinner: Roti made with whole wheat, soup, salad, rice, and dal

Conclusion:

Numerous nations have been affected by the obesity epidemic, which is still expanding at an alarming rate. The rising pattern has been seen across numerous populaces and age bunches including the old, the young, kids, grown-ups, men, youths, and ladies of child-bearing age. The medical and quality of life effects of obesity are numerous, and obesity is a serious threat to public health. Anecdotal accounts of the effects of obesity are common and echoed by people who are obese. The negative effects of obesity on health and social life worry a lot of people. This audit can assist with bringing issues to light on the well-being and personal satisfaction results of corpulence. Increased interest in obesity treatment and prevention can result from raising awareness of these effects. It might likewise rouse and urge individuals to lose abundant weight to work on their well-being and personal satisfaction. For those who are currently complacent about their dietary caloric intake and their excess body weight, public health education, open discussion, and awareness of the negative effects of obesity can act as a deterrent and/or a wake-up call. Bringing issues to light may likewise prod people in general into it. The obesity epidemic and its consequences can be reduced through appropriate interventions and collaborative efforts by individuals, health professionals, businesses, and the government.

www.ingramcontent.com/pod-product-compliance
Lightning Source LLC
Chambersburg PA
CBHW061548250726
48657CB00006B/2366